POLYCYSTIC OVARY SYNDROME DIET COOKBOOK (PCOS)

Free 100 Diet Recipes and Their Preparation Procedures

Nutritional Delicacies and Lifestyle Changes To Manage PCOS Symptoms Naturally

Dr. Marley Marian

Table of Contents

Chapter One

Introduction

Polycystic Ovary Syndrome (PCOS) affects millions of women worldwide, presenting with a complicated set of symptoms that may have a substantial effect on health and quality of life.

This disorder, which is characterized by hormonal imbalance, insulin resistance, and reproductive difficulties, necessitates multifaceted management measures for optimal therapy. Nutrition is one of the most important measures for relieving symptoms and boosting general well-being.

In this discussion, we will look at the complexities of PCOS, including its etiology, symptoms, and the critical role diet plays in controlling the illness. We also include a selected selection of 100 recipes designed particularly to help with PCOS control, as well as preparation instructions.

Understanding PCOS

Polycystic Ovarian Syndrome (PCOS) is a hormonal condition that mostly affects women of reproductive age. It is characterized by irregular menstrual periods, high testosterone levels, and ovarian cysts. Despite the term, not all women with PCOS have ovarian cysts, and not all ovarian cysts indicate PCOS.

What Is Polycystic Ovarian Syndrome?

PCOS is a complex illness that includes genetics, insulin resistance, and hormone abnormalities. Women with PCOS often have irregular or nonexistent menstrual cycles, excessive hair growth, acne, weight gain, and reproductive difficulties. These symptoms might vary in intensity across people, making diagnosis and treatment difficult.

Causes Of PCOS

The actual etiology of PCOS is unknown; however various variables are thought to contribute to its development. Genetics plays an important role since women with a family history of PCOS are more likely to acquire the illness. Insulin resistance, in which the body's cells do not react properly to insulin, is another typical symptom of PCOS. This causes high insulin levels, which stimulates the ovaries to create extra androgens like testosterone.

Symptoms Of PCOS

PCOS causes a wide variety of symptoms that might develop differently in each person. Common symptoms include irregular menstrual periods, hirsutism (excessive hair growth), acne, weight gain, and infertility. Furthermore, women with PCOS may suffer mood fluctuations, lethargy, and hair loss. The degree and mix of symptoms vary greatly amongst afflicted people.

Chapter Two

Importance Of Recipes For Managing PCOS And Preparation Procedures

Polycystic ovary syndrome (PCOS) is a hormonal condition that affects about one in every ten women of reproductive age worldwide. PCOS treatment is a complex strategy that includes lifestyle changes, medication, and nutritional alterations.

Among them, PCOS-specific recipes may be very beneficial. Here, we discuss the importance of such dishes and present a thorough list of 100 essential recipes for controlling PCOS, along with preparation instructions.

The Significance Of PCOS-Friendly Recipes

PCOS-friendly meals are intended to meet the dietary demands of people with PCOS by emphasizing nutrient-dense foods that help regulate blood sugar levels, control insulin resistance, and promote hormonal balance. These recipes often highlight complete, unprocessed meals and include elements believed to aid with PCOS control, such as lean meats, fiber-rich veggies, and healthy fats.

The Importance Of Preparation Procedures

The preparation techniques for PCOS-friendly dishes are equally important. Proper cooking procedures and techniques may retain the nutritional integrity of products while also increasing their bioavailability, guaranteeing the most benefit for those with PCOS. Furthermore, precise and simple preparation instructions make it easier for people to follow the recipes and integrate them into their everyday lives.

List Of 100 Essential Recipes For Managing PCOS

1. Quinoa Breakfast Bowl: Cook quinoa and top with berries, almonds, and honey for a healthy start to the day.

2. Salmon and Avocado Salad: Make a protein-rich salad with grilled salmon, avocado, lush greens, and light vinaigrette.

3. Chia Seed Pudding: Combine chia seeds, almond milk, and sweetener of choice, and then chill overnight for a wonderful and full dessert or breakfast.

4. Turkey and Vegetable Stir-Fry: Sauté lean turkey with mixed veggies and low-sodium soy sauce for a fast and tasty supper.

5. Sweet Potato and Black Bean Tacos: For a hearty vegetarian supper, fill whole-grain tortillas with roasted sweet potatoes, black beans, avocado, and salsa.

6. Greek Yogurt Parfait: Combine Greek yogurt, fresh fruit, and granola for a balanced and delicious snack.

7. Egg Muffins: Combine eggs, spinach, bell peppers, and feta cheese, then bake in muffin pans for a convenient and protein-rich breakfast.

8. Spiralize zucchini and combine it with homemade pesto for a low-carb twist on conventional pasta recipes.

9. Cauliflower Fried Rice: For a healthy spin on a takeaway classic, pulse cauliflower in a food processor before stir-frying with veggies, egg, and soy sauce.

10. Lean Ground Beef Chili: Cook lean ground beef with tomatoes, beans, and spices to make a substantial and filling chili.

11. Coconut Flour Pancakes: Replace regular flour with coconut flour to produce fluffy, gluten-free pancakes that are low in carbs.

12. Stuffed Bell Peppers: Stuff half bell peppers with quinoa, lean mince turkey, and veggies, then bake until soft for a healthful and colorful lunch.

13. Mediterranean Veggie Bowl: To make a Mediterranean-inspired dinner, combine roasted veggies, chickpeas, olives, and feta cheese with a lemon-herb sauce.

14. Cucumber Avocado Rolls: Combine cucumber slices, avocado, smoked salmon, and cream cheese to make a light and pleasant appetizer or snack.

15. Almond Flour Banana Bread: Combine almond flour and ripe bananas to create a moist and tasty banana bread that is rich in protein and low in carbohydrates.

16. Spinach & Feta Stuffed Chicken Breast: For a simple but beautiful supper, stuff chicken breasts with sautéed spinach and feta cheese before baking until cooked through.

17. Berry Smoothie Bowl: For a nutritious breakfast or snack, combine mixed berries, Greek yogurt, and a splash of almond milk, then top with granola, almonds, and seeds.

18. Lentil Soup: Combine lentils, veggies, and herbs to make a hearty and healthy soup rich in fiber and protein.

19. Tuna Salad Lettuce Wraps: Combine canned tuna, Greek yogurt, chopped veggies, and spices; wrap in lettuce leaves for a light and protein-rich lunch.

20. Vegetable Frittata: Combine eggs, different veggies, and cheese, then bake until set for a flexible and fulfilling dish that can be served at any time of day.

21. Cauliflower Pizza Crust: Combine cauliflower florets, eggs, and cheese to create a gluten-free, low-carb pizza crust that can be topped with your favorite toppings.

22. Stuffed Portobello Mushrooms: For a vegetarian lunch, fill portobello mushroom caps with quinoa, spinach, and feta cheese before baking until golden and bubbling.

23. Oatmeal Banana Cookies: Combine ripe bananas, oats, almonds, and cinnamon, then bake for a healthy and naturally sweet dessert.

24. Chicken and Vegetable Skewers: Thread marinated chicken breast and veggies onto skewers, then grill until charred and thoroughly cooked for a tasty and colorful feast.

25. Butternut Squash Soup: Roast butternut squash until soft, then purée with broth, spices, and a splash of cream to make a creamy, warming soup.

26. Shrimp and Veggie Stir-Fry: Sauté shrimp with bell peppers, broccoli, and snap peas in a tasty sauce for a fast and nutritious midweek supper.

27. Quinoa Stuffed Peppers: Fill bell peppers with cooked quinoa, black beans, corn, and salsa, then bake until soft for a filling and protein-packed dinner.

28. Avocado Egg Salad: Combine avocado, hard-boiled eggs, mustard, and spices to make a creamy and healthful variation on conventional egg salad.

29. Turkey Meatballs: Combine ground turkey, breadcrumbs, herbs, and spices; bake until golden brown for a lean and tasty protein choice.

30. Cottage Cheese Pancakes: Mix cottage cheese, eggs, and oat flour to produce protein-packed pancakes that are light and fluffy.

31. Vegetable and Lentil Curry: Cook lentils and veggies in a fragrant curry sauce to make a substantial and fulfilling vegetarian supper.

32. Salmon patties: Combine canned salmon, breadcrumbs, herbs, and egg, then pan-fry until golden brown for a tasty and omega-3-rich alternative to beef patties.

33. Eggplant wrap-Ups: For a vegetarian Italian-inspired meal, roast eggplant slices then wrap them up with ricotta cheese and marinara sauce before baking until bubbling.

34. Chickpea Salad: Combine cooked chickpeas, diced vegetables, herbs, and a lemon-tahini dressing to make a pleasant and protein-rich salad.

35. Turkey Chili: Cook ground turkey with tomatoes, beans, and spices to make a lighter and leaner version of traditional chili.

36. Broccoli & Cheddar Frittata: Combine eggs, steamed broccoli, and shredded cheddar cheese, then bake until puffed and golden for a quick and filling supper.

37. Cauliflower Tabbouleh: For a grain-free take on classic tabbouleh salad, pulse cauliflower in a food

processor before tossing it with parsley, mint, tomatoes, and lemon juice.

38. Zucchini Bread Oatmeal: Combine oats, grated zucchini, cinnamon, and vanilla for a healthful and warm breakfast.

39. Stuffed Acorn Squash: For a festive and savory side dish, fill roasted acorn squash halves with quinoa, dried cranberries, and walnuts before baking until cooked through.

40. Caprese Salad: For a simple yet elegant appetizer or side dish, layer sliced tomatoes, fresh mozzarella, and basil leaves. Drizzle with balsamic sauce.

41. Turkey & Vegetable Meatloaf: Combine ground turkey, shredded veggies, and seasonings, then bake until well-cooked for a lean and tasty take on conventional meatloaf.

42. Mushroom Risotto: Sauté mushrooms with arborio rice, garlic, and white wine before simmering in broth till creamy and soft for a rich and comfortable meal.

43. Cauliflower Alfredo Pasta: Combine steamed cauliflower, garlic, Parmesan cheese, and milk to create a creamy, guilt-free Alfredo sauce for pasta.

44. Stuffed Cabbage Rolls: For a delicious and comfortable supper, stuff blanched cabbage leaves with ground turkey, rice, and marinara sauce. Bake until soft.

45. Sweet Potato Meal Hash: Sauté chopped sweet potatoes, onions, bell peppers, and turkey sausage for a colorful and substantial meal.

46. Salmon and Asparagus Foil Packets: Bake seasoned salmon fillets and asparagus stalks in foil until soft and flaky for a quick and nutritious supper.

47. Quinoa Black Bean Salad: Combine cooked quinoa, black beans, corn, tomatoes, avocado, and lime vinaigrette to make a delicious and protein-rich salad.

48. Eggplant Parmesan: For a lighter and vegetarian version of this famous Italian meal, bread and bake eggplant slices before layering them with marinara sauce and mozzarella.

49. Chicken and Vegetable Soup: Combine chicken breast, veggies, herbs, and stock to make a soothing and healthy soup ideal for cold days.

50. Cauliflower Mash: Steam cauliflower until soft, then purée with garlic, butter, and milk for a velvety, low-carb substitute for mashed potatoes.

51. Stuffed Bell Pepper Soup: Make a substantial and flavorful soup by simmering bell peppers, ground turkey, rice, and tomatoes in stock.

52. Vegetable and Bean Chili: Combine various veggies and beans with tomatoes and spices to make a hearty and nourishing vegetarian chili.

53. Turkey & Spinach Lasagna: For a lighter and more protein-packed take on this traditional Italian meal, layer cooked lasagna noodles with ground turkey, spinach, ricotta, and marinara sauce.

54. Cauliflower Rice Stir-Fry: Sauté cauliflower rice with veggies, egg, and soy sauce to make a low-carb and tasty alternative to classic rice meals.

55. Greek Turkey Burgers: Combine ground turkey, feta cheese, spinach, and Greek spices, then grill until thoroughly cooked for a tasty and protein-rich burger choice.

56. Stuffed Mushroom Caps: For a flavorful and fulfilling appetizer, fill mushroom caps with cream cheese, herbs, and breadcrumbs before baking until brown and bubbling.

57. Turkey & Sweet Potato Skillet: Cook ground turkey with chopped sweet potatoes, onions, and bell peppers in a one-pan dish that is fast, simple, and healthful.

58. Cauliflower Buffalo Bites: For a healthier alternative to typical buffalo wings, coat cauliflower florets with buffalo sauce and breadcrumbs before baking until crispy.

59. Shrimp and Quinoa Salad: For a delicious and protein-packed salad, combine cooked quinoa, shrimp, cucumber, tomatoes, and feta cheese, then drizzle with a lemon-tahini vinaigrette.

60. Mushroom & Spinach Stuffed Chicken Breast: Fill chicken breasts with sautéed mushrooms, spinach, and goat cheese, then bake until golden and juicy for an elegant and savory supper.

61. Cauliflower Pizza Bagels: Create a creative and personalized take on conventional pizza by topping cauliflower pizza crusts with marinara sauce, cheese, and your favorite toppings.

62. Salmon and Vegetable Skewers: Thread salmon fillets and other vegetables onto skewers, then grill until the fish is cooked through and the veggies are soft for a tasty and nutritious lunch.

63. Turkey Taco Lettuce Wraps: Fill lettuce leaves with seasoned ground turkey, black beans, corn, and salsa for a light and protein-rich alternative to classic tacos.

64. Cauliflower Gnocchi: Combine the cauliflower rice, almond flour, egg, and spices to produce gluten-free, low-carb gnocchi that tastes great with marinara or pesto.

65. Stuffed Zucchini Boats: For a filling and healthy supper, hollow out zucchini halves and stuff with ground turkey, quinoa, and marinara sauce before baking until soft.

66. Mediterranean Stuffed Chicken Breast: For a tasty and elegant dinner, stuff chicken breasts with spinach, sun-dried tomatoes, and feta cheese before baking until golden and cooked through.

67. Cauliflower Tacos: Roast cauliflower florets with taco seasoning before serving in tortillas with avocado, salsa, and cilantro for a wonderful vegan taco alternative.

68. Turkey and Vegetable Soup: Combine ground turkey, veggies, stock, and herbs to make a substantial and warming soup ideal for meal prep or quick weekday meals.

69. Cauliflower Mac and Cheese: To make a creamy and cozy macaroni and cheese substitute, blend steamed cauliflower with cheese and milk before tossing it with cooked pasta.

70. Stuffed Bell Pepper Casserole: In a casserole dish, layer cooked quinoa, ground turkey, bell peppers, and marinara sauce. Bake until bubbling and golden for a filling and healthy dinner.

71. Greek Stuffed Peppers: Stuff bell peppers with minced turkey, rice, spinach, and feta cheese, then bake until soft for a tasty and protein-rich dinner.

72. Cauliflower Hummus: Combine cooked cauliflower, chickpeas, tahini, garlic, and lemon juice to make a creamy and healthy dip that goes well with raw veggies or whole-grain crackers.

73. Turkey & Vegetable Skillet: For a fast and healthy supper, sauté ground turkey with diced veggies and seasonings before serving overcooked quinoa or brown rice.

74. Cauliflower Shepherd's Pie: For a lighter and lower-carb take on this traditional comfort dish, top a combination of ground turkey and veggies with mashed cauliflower rather than mashed potatoes.

75. Mediterranean Turkey Meatballs: Combine ground turkey, garlic, herbs, and spices, then bake until golden brown. Serve with tzatziki sauce for a tasty and protein-packed appetizer or main meal.

76. Cauliflower Breadsticks: For a low-carb alternative to classic breadsticks, combine cauliflower, cheese, eggs, and spices. Bake until golden and crispy.

77. Turkey & Quinoa Stuffed Peppers: Stuff bell peppers with cooked quinoa, ground turkey, veggies, and cheese, then bake until soft for a healthy and filling supper.

78. Cauliflower Rice Burrito Bowl: For a nutritious and tasty burrito bowl, combine seasoned cauliflower rice, black beans, grilled chicken or tofu, avocado, salsa, and shredded cheese.

79. Greek Turkey Meatballs: Combine ground turkey, feta cheese, spinach, and Greek spices, then bake until golden brown. Serve with tzatziki sauce for a tasty and protein-rich meal.

80. Cauliflower Mashed Potatoes: For a low-carb alternative to typical mashed potatoes, combine cooked cauliflower, garlic, butter, and milk until smooth and creamy.

81. Turkey & Black Bean Tacos: Fill whole-grain tortillas with seasoned ground turkey, black beans, corn, and salsa for a simple and tasty weekday meal.

82. Cauliflower Fried "Rice": In a food processor, pulse cauliflower until it resembles rice, then stir-fry with veggies, egg, and soy sauce for a low-carb and healthful substitute for classic fried rice.

83. Mediterranean Turkey Burgers: Combine ground turkey, feta cheese, olives, and Greek spices; grill until cooked through. Serve on whole-grain buns with tzatziki sauce and cucumber slices.

84. Cauliflower Breaded Chicken: For a healthier alternative to standard breaded chicken, coat chicken breasts in seasoned cauliflower breadcrumbs and bake until golden and crispy.

85. Turkey & Quinoa Meatballs: Combine ground turkey, cooked quinoa, herbs, and spices, then bake until golden brown. Serve with marinara sauce for a tasty and protein-packed meal.

86. Cauliflower Grits: Blend cooked cauliflower with cheese, butter, and milk until smooth and creamy, then serve as a low-carb substitute for regular grits.

87. Turkey & Black Bean Chili: Combine ground turkey, black beans, tomatoes, and spices to make a substantial and filling chili ideal for meal prep or warm weekday meals.

88. Cauliflower Pizza: For a gluten-free and low-carb alternative to regular pizza, start with cauliflower pizza dough and top with your favorite pizza toppings.

89. Turkey and Vegetable Stir-Fry: Sauté ground turkey with veggies and soy sauce before serving over cooked quinoa or brown rice for a simple and healthy midweek supper.

90. Cauliflower potato Tots: For a healthy alternative to classic potato tots, combine cauliflower, cheddar, egg, and spices before shaping into tots and baking until golden and crispy.

91. Turkey & Sweet Potato Hash: Sauté ground turkey with chopped sweet potatoes, onions, and bell peppers before topping with a fried egg for a substantial breakfast or brunch.

92. Cauliflower Gnocchi with Pesto: For a tasty and healthy supper, combine cooked cauliflower gnocchi with homemade pesto sauce and grated Parmesan cheese.

93. Turkey & Vegetable Skillet: Sauté mince turkey with diced veggies and Italian seasoning before serving overcooked pasta or spaghetti squash for a simple and savory supper.

94. Cauliflower "Fried Rice": In a food processor, pulse cauliflower until it resembles rice, then stir-fry with veggies, egg, and soy sauce for a low-carb and healthful substitute for classic fried rice.

95. Turkey & Black Bean Stuffed Peppers: Stuff bell peppers with ground turkey, black beans, corn, and salsa, then bake until soft for a tasty and protein-rich dinner.

96. Cauliflower dough Pizza: For a gluten-free and low-carb alternative to regular pizza, start with cauliflower pizza dough and top with your favorite pizza toppings.

97. Turkey & Quinoa Stuffed Bell Peppers: Stuff bell peppers with cooked quinoa, ground turkey, veggies, and cheese, then bake until soft for a healthy and filling dinner.

98. Cauliflower Alfredo Sauce: For a lighter and healthier version of conventional Alfredo sauce, blend cooked cauliflower with garlic, Parmesan cheese, and milk until smooth and creamy before tossing over cooked pasta.

99. Turkey and Vegetable Soup: Combine ground turkey, veggies, stock, and herbs to make a substantial and warming soup ideal for meal prep or quick weekday meals.

100. Cauliflower Rice Stir-Fry: Sauté cauliflower rice with veggies, egg, and soy sauce to make a low-carb and tasty alternative to classic rice meals.

To summarize, PCOS-friendly meals are useful tools for controlling PCOS symptoms while also improving overall health and wellness. Individuals with PCOS may enjoy a broad range of tasty and gratifying meals that meet their specific dietary requirements by adding nutrient-dense products and following suitable cooking practices.

From breakfast to supper and everything in between, this varied collection of recipes provides inspiration and assistance for making healthful and delectable foods that contribute to a balanced and sustainable approach to PCOS treatment.

Chapter Three

10 Snacks For PCOS Management

1. Greek yogurt with strawberries and almonds

2. Sliced apples and almond butter

3. Carrot sticks and hummus

4. Hard-boiled eggs.

5. Cottage cheese with pineapple chunks

6. Edamame

7. Mixed nut and dried fruit

8. Celery sticks and peanut butter

9. Cherry tomatoes with mozzarella cheese

10. Avocado on Whole Grain Toast

10 Smoothies For PCOS Management

1. Berry Blast Smoothie contains spinach, mixed berries, Greek yogurt, almond milk, and flaxseeds.

2. Green Goddess Smoothie contains kale, pineapple, banana, avocado, and coconut water.

3. Tropical Paradise Smoothie contains mango, banana, coconut milk, spinach, and chia seeds.

4. Peanut Butter Banana Smoothie contains bananas, peanut butter, oats, almond milk, and honey.

5. Chocolate Avocado Smoothie contains avocado, chocolate powder, banana, almond milk, and honey.

6. Berry Spinach Smoothie contains spinach, mixed berries, Greek yogurt, almond milk, and hemp seeds.

7. Mango Tango Smoothie contains mango, orange juice, Greek yogurt, spinach, and flaxseed.

8. Peachy Green Smoothie contains peaches, spinach, banana, almond milk, and chia seeds.

9. Blueberry Almond Smoothie contains blueberries, almond butter, Greek yogurt, almond milk, and oats.

10. Pumpkin Spice Smoothie contains pumpkin puree, banana, cinnamon, almond milk, and vanilla protein powder.

Incorporating these snacks and smoothies into your diet will help control PCOS symptoms while also delivering important nutrients for general health and well-being. To maximize PCOS management and increase quality of life, remember to eat complete foods, lean proteins, healthy fats, and stay hydrated.

The Consequences Of Untreated PCOS

PCOS often remains undetected or untreated, resulting in a variety of health issues. Untreated PCOS may have serious repercussions, affecting both physical and mental well-being. Here are ten severe problems that patients may suffer if PCOS is left untreated:

1. Irregular Menstrual periods: One of the most common symptoms of PCOS is irregular menstrual periods, which may make conception difficult and cause reproductive complications.

2. Increased Risk of Infertility: PCOS is one of the primary reasons for infertility in women, owing to irregular or absent ovulation.

3. Weight Gain and Obesity: Insulin resistance, which is usually linked with PCOS, often causes weight gain and obesity, compounding hormonal imbalances and raising the risk of various health issues such as type 2 diabetes and cardiovascular disease.

4. High Androgen Levels: PCOS may induce an increase in androgens (male hormones), resulting in acne, hirsutism (excessive hair growth), and male pattern baldness.

5. Metabolic Syndrome: People with untreated PCOS are more likely to develop metabolic syndrome, which is defined by a group of disorders such as high blood pressure, high blood sugar, extra abdominal fat, and abnormal cholesterol levels.

6. Type 2 Diabetes: Insulin resistance is a common symptom of PCOS and may lead to type 2 diabetes if not treated.

7. Women with PCOS are more likely to develop cardiovascular disorders such as heart disease, stroke, and hypertension, which are caused in part by obesity, insulin resistance, and dyslipidemia.

8. Endometrial Cancer: In women with PCOS, irregular menstrual cycles and unopposed estrogen exposure owing to a lack of ovulation increase the risk of endometrial hyperplasia and endometrial cancer.

9. Mental Health Issues: PCOS has been linked to an increased incidence of anxiety, depression, and mood disorders, all of which may have a negative influence on quality of life if not addressed.

10. Reduced Quality of Life: If the physical symptoms, reproductive issues, and mental anguish associated with PCOS are not handled properly, the overall quality of life may suffer.

PCOS And Diet: An Overview

Diet has an important role in controlling PCOS symptoms and lowering the risk of complications. A well-balanced diet may help control insulin levels, manage weight, and improve overall health outcomes for those with PCOS.

The Impact Of Lifestyle Changes

In addition to food adjustments, lifestyle improvements such as regular exercise, stress management, and proper sleep are critical components of PCOS treatment. These adjustments may assist in enhancing insulin sensitivity, managing hormonal balance, and relieving symptoms.

Understanding Insulin Resistance In PCOS

Insulin resistance is a major underlying element in PCOS pathophysiology, causing a variety of metabolic and reproductive problems. treating insulin resistance with food, exercise, and medication is critical to properly treating PCOS symptoms.

Chapter Four

Glycemic Index And PCOS

Foods having a high glycemic index might worsen insulin resistance and should be avoided in the diet of people with PCOS. Low glycemic index meals may help regulate blood sugar and enhance insulin sensitivity.

Importance Of Regular Exercise

Regular exercise is essential for PCOS treatment because it improves insulin sensitivity, helps with weight control, reduces stress, and regulates menstrual cycles. Here are some reasons why exercise is essential for people with PCOS.

1. Increased insulin sensitivity

2. Weight management

3. Hormonal Balance

4. Regulation of menstrual cycle

5. Reduced androgen levels

6. Higher energy levels

7. Improved mood and mental wellbeing

8. Reduced risk of cardiovascular illnesses.

9. Improved fertility

10. Better overall health results.

Stress Management Strategies for PCOS

Stress may aggravate PCOS symptoms by causing hormonal imbalances and increasing insulin resistance. Stress management practices such as mindfulness, meditation, yoga, and relaxation exercises may help relieve symptoms and enhance overall quality of life.

Key Nutrients to Manage PCOS Symptoms

Certain nutrients are essential for treating PCOS symptoms and improving overall health. Here are ten essential nutrients that people with PCOS should emphasize in their diet:

1.Omega-3 Fatty Acids

2. Chromium

3. Magnesium

4. Vitamin D

5. Inositol

6. Zinc

7. B vitamins (particularly B12 and folate)

8. Iron

9. Calcium

10. Fiber

Meal Plan for PCOS

Effective meal planning includes selecting nutrient-dense meals that support hormonal balance, manage blood sugar levels, and improve general health. Including a mix of fruits, vegetables, lean meats, whole grains, and healthy fats in meals may help people with PCOS manage their symptoms more efficiently.

Planning A PCOS-Friendly Diet

A PCOS-friendly diet emphasizes complete, unprocessed foods, low glycemic index carbs, enough protein, and healthy fats while limiting added sugars and refined carbohydrates. Individuals might benefit from consulting with a qualified dietitian to create individualized meal plans based on their unique requirements and objectives.

Individuals with PCOS may successfully manage their symptoms, enhance their quality of life, and lower their risk of long-term issues by taking a comprehensive strategy that includes food, lifestyle changes, and medication therapies.

Meal Time And Frequency For PCOS

Polycystic Ovary Syndrome (PCOS) is a hormonal condition that mostly affects women of reproductive age, resulting in irregular menstrual periods, elevated testosterone levels, and polycystic ovaries. While addressing PCOS requires a variety of strategies, including medication and lifestyle modifications, paying attention to meal time and frequency is critical for symptom management and general health.

Meal Timing: Women with PCOS might benefit from eating breakfast within an hour of waking up. This helps to control blood sugar levels and jumpstart metabolism for the day. According to research, women with PCOS may have poor glucose tolerance and insulin resistance, thus it is critical to spread meals out evenly throughout the day to minimize blood sugar spikes and falls.

Intermittent fasting, which includes alternating between eating and fasting intervals, has grown in popularity due to possible health advantages such as better insulin sensitivity. However, for women with PCOS, intermittent fasting should be approached with caution.

Some people may find it beneficial, while others may notice negative effects on hormone balance and menstrual regularity. It is recommended that you consult with a healthcare practitioner or a licensed nutritionist before commencing intermittent fasting.

Eating Out With PCOS

Maintaining a PCOS-friendly diet when dining out might be difficult, but not impossible. With careful decisions and techniques, it is feasible to enjoy eating out without jeopardizing one's health objectives.

Menu Selection: When eating out, choose restaurants that have a range of entire foods, such as grilled lean meats, salads with dressing on the side, and vegetable-based sides. Avoid foods that are deep fried, excessively sauced, or high in processed carbs and sugars.

Portion Control: Restaurant servings are often bigger than required, which leads to overeating. To prevent this, try splitting a meal with a dining companion, ordering an appetizer or half portions, or requesting a to-go box at the start of the dinner to divide out leftovers.

Social gatherings and activities often focus on food, making it difficult for those with PCOS to keep to their dietary plans. However, with little preparation and mental changes, it is feasible to manage social settings while controlling PCOS.

Communication: Informing friends and family about your dietary choices and health objectives might help reduce the urge to eat items that aggravate PCOS symptoms. When people understand why others make certain food choices, they are more likely to be understanding and accommodating.

Healthy swaps: When attending social occasions with food, bring PCOS-friendly meals to share. This guarantees that there are alternatives accessible that meet dietary requirements while yet allowing for group meal experiences.

Healthy Cooking Techniques For PCOS

The cooking techniques employed may have a considerable influence on the nutritional content of meals, thus it is important to choose ways that maintain nutrients while limiting the addition of bad fats and sugar.

Grilling and roasting are wonderful ways of cooking lean meats and vegetables that give an exquisite taste without the use of excessive oils or fats. Marinades created with herbs, citrus juices, and spices may boost taste without adding extra calories or sugar.

Steaming and boiling are moderate cooking techniques that assist in preserving the inherent nutrients in foods like vegetables, seafood, and grains. These approaches need little extra lipids and might be especially effective for PCOS patients aiming to control their weight and insulin levels.

Chapter Five

Planning meals ahead of time may help people with PCOS make better choices and stick to regular eating habits, which can improve hormone balance and general health.

Sample breakfast options include a spinach and mushroom omelet with whole grain bread, Greek yogurt with berries and nuts, and overnight oats with almond milk, chia seeds, and sliced fruit.

Sample lunch options include grilled chicken salad with avocado and balsamic vinaigrette, quinoa salad with roasted vegetables and lemon-tahini dressing, and turkey and hummus wrap with raw veggies sticks.

Sample dinner options include baked fish with broccoli and quinoa, stir-fried tofu with veggies in ginger-soy sauce over brown rice, and zucchini noodles with marinara sauce and turkey meatballs.

Creating A Supportive Environment For PCOS Management.

When dealing with PCOS, having support from family, friends, and healthcare professionals is vital. Creating a supportive atmosphere may help people remain motivated, responsible, and empowered while making beneficial lifestyle choices.

Education and Awareness: Educating loved ones about PCOS and its symptoms may help them understand and empathize, making it simpler to make dietary and lifestyle adjustments. Encouraging open communication and giving opportunities for more learning may help support networks provide real assistance.

Encouragement and accountability: Regular check-ins and encouragement from supporting people may help people with PCOS keep motivated and on track to achieve their health objectives. Whether it's an exercise companion, a cooking partner, or a supportive friend, having someone to share accomplishments and problems with may make a big difference in long-term adherence to healthy behaviors.

Tracking Progress And Making Adjustments

Monitoring progress and making changes as required are critical components of effective PCOS treatment. Tracking several elements of health, such as nutritional consumption, physical activity, and symptom severity, may give useful information and help guide decision-making.

Food Journaling: Keeping a food diary may help people with PCOS discover trends and causes for their symptoms. Meals, snacks, and any related symptoms such as bloating, weariness, or mood swings may be tracked to identify links between nutrition and health outcomes.

Symptom Tracking: Tracking menstrual cycles, energy levels, and mood swings may give useful information for learning how lifestyle variables such as nutrition and exercise affect PCOS symptoms. Apps and internet tools may help expedite symptom monitoring and spot patterns over time.

To summarize, successful PCOS management involves meal timing and frequency, handling social circumstances, healthy cooking techniques, sample meal planning, providing a supportive atmosphere, and evaluating progress. Individuals with PCOS may improve their health, and reduce symptoms, and general quality of life by implementing these measures into their everyday lives.

Keeping Motivated On Your PCOS Diet Journey

Living with Polycystic Ovary Syndrome (PCOS) may provide unique problems, especially in terms of nutrition and lifestyle. From overcoming food cravings to overcoming setbacks and staying motivated, the path to improved health with PCOS involves effort and determination. However, equipped with information and techniques, you can remain on track and reach your health objectives. In this comprehensive guide, we'll go over key aspects of staying motivated on your PCOS diet journey, such as understanding food cravings, dealing with setbacks, incorporating mindful eating practices, recognizing the value of sleep, addressing fertility concerns, managing PCOS during pregnancy, postpartum management, and concluding with essential author appreciation.

Understanding Food Cravings And PCOS

Individuals with PCOS encounter considerable difficulty in regulating food desires, which may be impacted by hormonal abnormalities and insulin resistance. Understanding the underlying causes of these urges is critical for devising effective measures to address them.

High insulin levels in the body, which are often related to PCOS, may cause increased appetite and cravings for sweet and high-carbohydrate meals. Additionally, variations in hormones such as leptin and ghrelin may aggravate desires, making it harder to stick to a balanced diet.

Chapter Six

Dealing with Setbacks

Setbacks are a normal part of any journey, including treating PCOS. Setbacks, whether they be due to poor food choices, missed workouts, or unanticipated weight gain, may be upsetting. However, it is critical to handle failures with compassion and resilience.

Instead of concentrating on errors, see them as learning opportunities. Reflect on what caused the setback and devise methods to avoid it from occurring again. Remember that development is not linear, and every setback provides a chance to recommit to your health objectives.

Implementing Mindful Eating Practices

Mindful eating entails paying attention to the current moment and completely engaged in the act of eating. This technique is especially good for those with PCOS since it increases awareness of hunger signals, satiety levels, and dietary choices. Slowing down and appreciating each meal will help you avoid overeating and make healthier food choices. Furthermore, practicing mindfulness may help decrease stress, which is critical for controlling PCOS symptoms.

The Significance Of Sleep In PCOS Management

Quality sleep is critical for general health and well-being, particularly in those with PCOS. Sleep deprivation may affect hormone levels, such as insulin, cortisol, and leptin, resulting in increased appetites, weight gain, and insulin resistance.

Prioritizing sleep hygiene behaviors, such as sticking to a regular sleep schedule, developing a calming bedtime ritual, and improving your sleeping environment, may greatly improve sleep quality and aid with PCOS treatment.

PCOS And Fertility: Dietary And Lifestyle Options

Many people with PCOS suffer from infertility owing to irregular ovulation and hormonal imbalance. While medical interventions like fertility treatments may be required for some, maintaining a good diet and lifestyle may also improve reproductive results. Incorporating nutrient-dense diets, reducing stress, keeping a healthy weight, and participating in regular physical exercise are all important variables in promoting fertility in PCOS patients.

Managing PCOS During Pregnant

Pregnancy may provide particular concerns for those with PCOS, including an increased risk of gestational diabetes, hypertension, and miscarriage. However, with the right medical treatment and lifestyle changes, many women with PCOS may have healthy pregnancies.

Working closely with healthcare specialists, eating a balanced diet, being physically active, and monitoring blood sugar levels are all important for treating PCOS throughout pregnancy and protecting the health of both mother and baby.

Postpartum Management Of PCOS

Women with PCOS may encounter extra obstacles after giving birth, such as hormonal swings, weight gain, and difficulty nursing. It is important to focus on self-care during the postpartum time and gradually resume healthy behaviors.

Gentle exercise, decent food, proper sleep, and assistance from healthcare experts and support groups may all help women navigate the postpartum period and successfully manage PCOS.

Conclusion

Managing PCOS requires a comprehensive strategy that includes dietary adjustments, lifestyle alterations, and self-care activities. Individuals may empower themselves by knowing the particular issues related to PCOS and developing ways to solve them. Remember that development may be gradual and nonlinear, but every tiny step forward helps you achieve your objectives.

Author Appreciation

I give Special appreciation to other writers and researchers for devoting their time and skills to researching PCOS, and contributing significant insights into its treatment. Your efforts have enabled many others to manage their PCOS journeys with knowledge, resilience, and hope.